Scabies Natural Home Treatment Solution

By: Alyson Rodgers

Disclaimer

This book is intended as a reference material, not as a medical manual to replace the advice of your physician or to substitute for any treatment prescribed by your physician.

If you are ill or suspect that you have a medical problem, we strongly encourage you to consult your medical, health, or other competent professional before adopting any of the suggestions in this book or drawing inferences from it. If you are taking prescription medication, you should never change your diet (for better or worse) without consulting your physician, as any dietary change may affect the metabolism of that prescription drug.

This book and the author's opinions are solely for informational and educational purposes.

The author specifically disclaims all responsibility for any liability, loss, or risk, personal or otherwise which is incurred as a consequence, directly or indirectly, of the use and application of any of the contents of this book. Individual results may vary.

Published by:
www.SparrowPublication.com
Alyson Rodgers and Random Technologies
4409 HOFFNER AVENUE, SUITE 347
Belle Isle, FL 32812

TABLE OF CONTENTS

IV. Traditional Solutions

    A. Prescription Options

        1. *Permethrin*

        2. *Crotamiton*

        3. *Ivermectin*

        4. *Malathion*

        5. *Lindane*

    B. Over-the-Counter Treatments

        1. *Permethrin*

        2. *Benzyl Benzoate*

V. Pharmaceuticals and their Issues

    A. *Pyrethrum*

    B. *Lindane*

    C. *Ivermectin*

    D. *Malathion*

    E. Additional Scabies Treatment Solutions

VI. Natural Scabies Treatments

    A. Herbal Solutions Guidelines

    B. Sulfur Cream

Introduction

Having scabies is exasperating; those who suffer from this parasitic malady are often by turns embarrassed and frustrated. When people develop scabies, they may not know that it is an infection caused by the mite *Sarcoptes scabiei*. They also may not know how the disease is transmitted or how to treat it.

People mistakenly believe that, because they

contracted mites, their personal hygiene is to blame. However, anyone can get scabies if he or she is exposed to someone who is already infested. Scabies is much like lice or even bedbugs, two similar conditions discussed later in this guide.

To be sure, there is no shortage of myths regarding scabies, as will be seen. This report tells the reader facts about this disease - how scabies is contracted and transmitted and the treatment options available. Included here are both conventional and natural regimens to combat this debilitating condition. Also considered are strategies to prevent an outbreak from spreading through a family's household.

Knowledge is power – This report will empower the reader with the knowledge needed to make the best decision about scabies treatment. Let the reader arm himself with the information below.

Facts about Scabies

Most people know little about scabies until they or someone they know becomes infested. Some may have heard of mange, which is the type of scabies that infects dogs, but often they do not know that humans are susceptible to a similar condition.

This is the first misconception about scabies: while similar, scabies and mange are different. Nobody gets scabies from dogs and dogs cannot contract mange from people. Either Demodex canus mite or the Sarcoptes scabiei canis mite causes mange.

What is Scabies?
Scabies is an infestation of the skin by the microscopic mite known by its Latin name *Sarcoptes scabei*. This infestation is common, found worldwide and can affect people of all races and social classes. Scabies spreads rapidly under crowded conditions where there is frequent skin-to-skin contact between people, such as in hospitals, penal institutions, child-care facilities, and nursing homes.

What a Scabies Mite is?
Scabies mites are not visible to the naked eye. They are arthropods, related to spiders and ticks. They have 8 jointed legs and are about the size of the period at the end of this sentence.

Most other mites feed on a variety of creatures in a variety of places but scabies mites are known for infesting their mammal host. When talking about scabies, "outside of the host" refers to the surface of the skin as well as burrowing into the skin. The scabies mite does not attack organs or reach the bloodstream.

They are very small, eyeless and somewhat turtle-shaped (flat on one side and curved on the other). They are usually white or clear.

Scabies Mite Life Cycle

Female mites usually live about a month, males somewhat less. Males are sexually mature in 10 days while females reach sexual maturity in 14 days. Female mites lay eggs from which larvae emerge after three or four days.

A female mite can lay two or three eggs daily while she is sexually mature (about two weeks) before death, totaling 28 to 42 eggs. Some reports say that as many as 90 percent of those potential mites will die before they reach maturity.

While in the human body, adult mites can burrow the length of their body daily or about a centimeter in their lifetime. Burrows are horizontal and sometimes visible on the victim's skin.

Scabies Effect on Human Skin

Scabies mites burrow into the skin using their mouths and front legs. They do not actually carry disease, but their presence in the body creates an immune system response called scabies.

Scabies usually manifests itself as a rash or pimple-like irritation at the site of infestation. The spots are itchy and the victim may contract infected sores from scratching the affected areas.

Rashes are often located between the fingers, in the fold of the elbow or knee, the armpit and genital regions.

How is Scabies Contracted?

Scabies is caused by direct, prolonged contact with an infected person. Another common misconception is that because scabies sores can be found on the hands, scabies is easily spread by shaking an infested person's hand.

While it is possible to contract scabies in this manner, it is highly unlikely. A mite would have to be on the surface of a person's skin, crawling onto the uninfected person, in order to infest him.

Mites can crawl about an inch a minute, so people who shake hands or embrace for an extended time could spread scabies. Intimate contact or sleeping next to someone with scabies is a much more likely scenario for transmission.

Scabies mites cannot jump, so by just being present in the

same room with someone who has scabies does not mean that it will spread to someone uninfected.

It is also possible to get scabies from clothing or linens used by an infected person. Those who share a bed or use a towel with someone who has scabies may also become infected.

Mites can live on clothing, carpeting and other fabrics for 2 to 5 days under normal room temperature and humidity. If the room is cooler than 50° Fahrenheit or higher than 90% humidity, mites will thrive for longer periods.

Mites that infect a host tend to be less effective at burrowing, especially after the first day and if conditions in the room are warm and dry.

Scabies Risks?

Scabies is relatively non-discriminatory. Anyone exposed for an extended period to somebody with scabies - especially if he has prolonged physical contact or contact with linens, clothing or fabric furniture that the infected person has used - is likely to contract scabies. It has nothing to do with personal hygiene.

Still, people with impaired immune systems and the elderly are more susceptible to a more severe form of scabies known as crusted or Norwegian scabies. This type of scabies is caused by the presence of many more mites on the body than are present with standard scabies. The body's reaction is more severe, often causing somewhat crusty or flaky sores.

When Does Symptoms Appear?

For those who have never had scabies before, it might take 4 to 6 weeks for symptoms to appear. Otherwise, symptoms develop more quickly, usually within 1 to 4 days.

These are the averages, but there have been cases of new infestation appearing within a week of exposure while others seem to have taken as long as a year for symptoms to appear.

Symptoms of a Scabies Infestation.

The main symptom of a scabies infestation is itching. This is an allergic reaction to the mites and it may become worse at night or after a hot shower.

Likely areas include:
• Between the fingers;
• Around the wrist;
• Around the waist or belt line;
• The abdomen;
• The groin area;
• Underarms;
• The folds of the elbows and knees.

Children commonly show scabies irritation on their faces, the palms of the hands and soles of the feet as well.

Other symptoms include red rashes that may be bumpy.

Pus-filled lesions are also possible. Burrows of 1/8 to 1/2 inch may be visible but they are often hard to see.

The rashes and irritation spots are not necessarily the locations of the mite burrows.

It is possible to get a secondary infection, such as a staph infection, because of excessive scratching and infection of the sores.

Scabies Diagnosis

It is important to see a doctor if scabies symptoms are detected. A doctor can examine the rash and burrows before diagnosing scabies or another condition.

Skin scraping is another method used to look for mites in the skin. However, this is not always effective at diagnosing scabies since the average person with scabies has only between 5 and 50 mites. Thus, it is easy to get a false negative if the skin test is relied upon exclusively for diagnosis.

It may be necessary to take 4 to 6 scrapings to increase the odds of finding mites. There is no guarantee that, because mites are not found, scabies mites are absent. Visible burrows most likely hold mites.

Other Health Issues

Several other ailments have similar symptoms to a scabies outbreak. Thus, it is important to visit a doctor should these symptoms appear rather than relying on self-diagnosis.

Other conditions that may have similar rashes and bumps include:

- Allergies or contact dermatitis;
- Atopic dermatitis, a genetic hypersensitivity;
- Eczema;
- Inflammation of the hair follicles;
- Fungal infection;
- Impetigo, a bacterial infection;
- Insect bites;
- Hives;
- Folliculitis;
- Rosacea;
- Shingles;
- Lymphoma;
- Adverse drug reaction;
- Mycosis fungoides, a T-cell lymphoma that affects skin;
- Neurodermatitis, chronic flaky or scaly skin;
- Psoriasis;
- Syphilis;
- Ringworm;
- Vasculitis, inflammation of blood vessels.

Scabies Treatment

Treatment options are the focus of much of the remainder of this book. At this point, suffice to say that topical insecticidal creams or lotions are commonly prescribed. The lotion is applied and left on the body overnight, then washed away in the morning. It is important when using an insecticidal method to follow diligently the directions as specified by the manufacturer. It is possible to become seriously ill should an excessive amount be used or if the lotion is applied too often.

There are also some alternative, natural methods used to eradicate scabies that will be discussed at length later in the guide.

How Long Before Scabies Disappear?

Once treatment is started, the patient is no longer contagious. While itching may be present for several weeks, the patient will not be able to pass scabies to others after initial treatment has begun. The itching is a side effect of many conventional treatments for scabies and does not indicate the presence of scabies mites.

Keeping Scabies from Infecting Others

All people who occupy common living space, have sexual relations or share any other extended physical contact with someone infected with scabies should be treated at the same time as the patient.

All used bedding and clothing should be washed in hot water and dried in clothes dryer at its hottest setting. Any non-machine, washable items worn or slept on for a week or so before treatment should be sealed in a plastic bag for at least 7 days before being used again.

Symptoms of No Scabies Treatment

Scabies does not go away on its own. If left untreated, mites will continue to multiply and reproduce. This will lead to persistent irritation of the skin and, of course, will allow continued transmission of scabies to others.

Left untreated for long periods, scabies can become a systemic infection that may even be life threatening. Long-term scabies infection has been linked to rheumatic heart disease.

Traditional Solutions

This chapter will discuss common prescription and over-the-counter remedies used to treat scabies. For alternative and natural treatments, see chapter 4.

Prescription Options

Permethrin
A 5% permethrin cream, sold under the names Lyclear, Elimite and Acticin, is the most commonly prescribed treatment for scabies. The drug, which paralyzes and kills mites, is over 90% effective when used correctly.

Side effects of itching, stinging and burning are common and should not be considered as a failure of the treatment.

The cream should be applied to a clean body. Apply the cream over the entire body from the chin down, including the genitals and the soles of the feet. The cream should also be applied under the fingernails and toenails.

Scabies in facial areas is rare and usually only happens to babies and small children. If there are scabies sores on the face or scalp, these areas should be treated as well. Exercise extreme condition to keep the lotion away from eyes, nose and ears.

After application, take care not to rub off the cream for 8 to 14 hours. It should be reapplied to places such as the soles of feet if the patient stands or the hands if they are washed during the treatment period.

When treatment is completed, the cream should be showered off.

Crotamiton
A 10% solution of crotamiton, sold under the brand name Eurax, is between 50% and 70 % effective at eliminating scabies.

This cream should be massaged into the skin of the entire body. Treatment should be repeated after 24 hours and then the patient's body should be washed 48 hours after the second treatment.

Side effects can include itching, burning, stinging, and

rash and skin irritation. It should not be used on open sores. Its effectiveness and safety for children and pregnant women has not been tested.

Ivermectin
Sold as Sklice and Stromectol in the United States (Mectizan in Canada), ivermectin has not been approved by the U.S. Food and Drug Administration for the treatment of scabies but has been proven to be 90% to 95% effective.

This drug was originally developed to treat intestinal worms and river blindness. It apparently paralyzes and kills microfilariae; scabies mites are seemingly affected in the same manner.

It is an oral pill and is best for people who cannot use cream treatments, such as people in nursing homes or hospitals that, for example, are on ventilators or those who have large open sores or lesions.

The pill is effective with just 1 dose taken with 8 ounces of water for typical infestations of scabies; a 2-pill treatment is 95 % effective at eradicating more severe forms.

Side effects can include rash, itching, swelling and dizziness. The drug has not been tested on children who weigh less than 33 pounds. It has not been tested and is not recommended for women who are pregnant or may become pregnant because of birth defects caused in laboratory animals.

It is thought that the drug is safe to take while nursing, although it does transfer to the mother's milk.

Those who have bronchial asthma should not take ivermectin because it may increase breathing difficulties.

Malathion

Another common treatment is malathion, which can be purchased in cream form with or without a prescription (depending upon country). Malathion in a 0.5% solution is marketed as the prescription Ovide in the United States.

Like other cream treatments, malathion is applied to the entire body from the neck down. It remains on the body a full 24 hours before being washed away. This treatment period is longer than most other options.

It should not be used on children younger than 6 months of age and it should not be kept on the body longer than 24 hours because of the risk of overdose.

Malathion is commonly used as a treatment for head lice but can also be used for scabies as a last resort after other treatments have failed. It is smelly, highly flammable and can cause respiratory problems if inhaled so its use should be closely monitored.

Lindane

Once the most popular treatment for both scabies and lice (tiny insects that also live on the human body and are commonly found in the hair, though there are lice that live on other parts of the body as well), lindane is sometimes sold under the brand name Kwell and can be found in lotions and shampoos.

It is still available by prescription and is widely prescribed, but the Food and Drug Administration has warned that people can have serious side effects even when using the drug properly.

Seizures, which have been deadly, can happen if too much lindane is used or after a second treatment. People who used the drug correctly have also reported seizures. Especially susceptible are the elderly, children, and people who weigh less than 110 pounds.

Lindane lotion is now considered as a last resort treatment only, when all other options have been tried unsuccessfully or other treatments cannot be tolerated. Only enough lindane for 1 treatment is prescribed in order to reduce the chances of using too much or reapplying the lotion too soon.

Lindane should never be used by people with seizure disorders or by breastfeeding mothers. It should not be used as a first treatment option or if crusty/broken skin or dermatitis is diagnosed. It should never be used on babies.

Make sure the attending physician knows the medications the patient is taking, if the patient is pregnant or has any health problems such as AIDS, brain tumors, liver disease or diabetes. Other side effects can include itching, burning, dry skin and/or rash.

Over-The-Counter Treatments

Permethrin

Permethrin is now available over-the-counter as well as by prescription. It is sold under the brand name Elimite or Nix Dermal Cream. It is important to use the 5% solution.

Do not try to cure scabies with a 1% cream rinse solution (which is also sold under the brand name Nix, or other treatments intended for lice). These products do not have sufficient potency to kill scabies. Further, they are not to remain on the body any longer than 10 minutes. This period is too short for the product to be effective, even with sufficient potency.

Benzyl Benzoate

Another topical treatment, benzyl benzoate is available without a prescription. Directions must be followed carefully in order to prevent side effects. Apply this ester completely over a washed and clean body from the neck down for 24 hours.

It is not known to cause problems for pregnant or nursing women, but the manufacturers advise that pregnant women should only use it if necessary and that breast-feeding should be stopped while using the drug.

Overdose is a potential problem with this medication, especially if the directions are not followed or if too large a dose is used. Warning symptoms include blistering, crusting, oozing, itching or scaling skin. Loss of consciousness is possible.

Pharmaceuticals and their Issues

Most of the conventional treatments for scabies involve potentially dangerous and frightening drugs. These treatments involve use of neurotoxins that paralyze and kill scabies mites.

It is no wonder that there are many warnings regarding the use of these drugs. If they harm the nervous system of a bug, it is reasonable to assume that there are serious and adverse side effects for humans.

Knowledge is power. You should never blindly accept a treatment protocol simply because a doctor "knows best." Conduct due diligence and learn the available treatment options. Moreover, find out what ingredients are in the drugs a doctor recommends. Once a patient is armed with this information, then he or she can decide the best treatment approach.

Below is further information concerning the chemicals commonly used in scabies treatments.

Pyrethrum

Gardeners and botanists are likely familiar with pyrethrum as it is used as an insecticide. Permethrin is made from a synthetic form of pyrethrum, a toxin originally from chrysanthemums.

Pyrethrum is a nerve toxin and considered moderately toxic to humans, especially when inhaled or ingested. Some people are allergic to these chemicals.

Signs of overexposure to pyrethrum include dermatitis, tremors, headaches and vomiting as well as lung and liver problems. It is thought that some pyrethroids (synthetic pyrethrum) may be carcinogenic (cause cancer).

Some sources say that people sensitive to ragweed should not be exposed to pyrethrum. The chemical may have an adverse effect on the immune system. It has been implicated in cases of Multiple Chemical Sensitivity.

Lindane
The potential for seizures and death when using lindane has been mentioned. However, this harmful drug has a litany of worrisome qualities.

It remains in use as an insecticidal treatment for lumber as well as lice, mange and scabies treatments for humans and animals. Yet it is a powerful poison and just 1/2 of a tablespoon ingested can prove fatal to humans.

It is known as a blood poison and is thought to be a carcinogen. It can cause aplastic anemia (a precursor to leukemia) as well as problems with the liver, kidneys and bone marrow. It also accumulates in breast tissue. Lindane has been linked to a rise in non-Hodgkin's lymphoma (a type of cancer) in farmers who use it on livestock and grain.

Lindane is associated with an increase in leukemia in children exposed to it as treatment for lice or scabies or as a pesticide.

Its use has been completely banned in more than 40 countries. Another 20 nations have severely restricted it and its use is banned for farming in the European Union. In the United States, agricultural use of lindane ended in 2007 and its use in medications is now limited to "second-line" treatments when other protocols have failed. California banned pharmaceutical lindane in 2002.

Ivermectin
Ivermectin is used as a treatment for worms in animals and it is well documented that overdoses can be fatal in domestic and farm animals. It has also been suggested that use of this drug can be fatal in humans. In one study, a nursing home ward found a significant increase in deaths when patients were treated with the drug.

Malathion
Malathion is another powerful insecticide that is used by farmers and some cities to control mosquito, boll weevil and fruit fly populations in their communities. It is a very powerful chemical.

Overexposure to malathion can cause headaches, nausea, dizziness, drowsiness, muscle weakness, difficulty breathing, diarrhea, confusion, blurred vision and even death when ingested.

The Environmental Protection Agency (EPA) recently revised its risk assessment on malathion, emphasizing that infants and children are 10 times more susceptible to malathion exposure compared to adults. Yet the EPA considers additional exposure to malathion by using Ovide (a medicinal preparation of malathion) does not pose an increased risk to even children. Still, it is considered "slightly toxic" and has been shown to cause birth and developmental defects in rats although scientists say such problems in humans are not likely under normal circumstances.

Additional Scabies Treatment Solutions
Naturally, many balk at dosing their family with pesticides that have potentially dangerous effects. What other options are available to eliminate scabies? Many natural methods work safely and effectively to eliminate scabies, as shown below.

Natural Scabies Treatments

Lately the medical community has begun to reconsider standard medical treatments for scabies. It seems that scabies mites are becoming immune to these commonly used treatments.

One reason? Drugs are used improperly - as when people use a 1% solution of permethrin when a 5% dose is needed. The mites that survive the treatment are stronger than before and thus become resistant to higher doses.

Whatever the cause, scabies mites do seem to be becoming resistant to the common drugs used to treat them. That means that alternative methods must be developed to eliminate scabies.

While no one finds super bugs a cause to celebrate, the fact that people are turning to other methods for treating scabies is a positive development. Since natural remedies are safer and gentler, they are a preferred treatment option compared to toxic drugs commonly used to treat scabies. Here are some effective natural methods and information on how they can be used.

Herbal Solutions Guidelines

Overall, herbal remedies are much safer than prescription drugs and have proven to be quite effective. This is not to say that they cannot cause harm. Certain herbs should not be taken while pregnant. Others can interact adversely with other medications and herbs.

Those who are inexperienced with herbs and natural remedies should consult knowledgeable advisers such as a naturopath, a trusted friend or herbal textbook.

Always follow the directions included with any pills, lotions, creams or tinctures. Recommendations given below are to be considered as guidelines only and are not intended as medical advice. The Food and Drug Administration does not evaluate herbal remedies, including single herbs and natural remedy blends designed to treat certain ailments. Thus, there is no guarantee as to the potency or effectiveness of any given product.

If more information is needed about any of the herbal remedies discussed, visit some of the web resources listed at the end of this guide or consult someone with knowledge of herbal remedies who can make recommendations for specific situations.

Many of these remedies are helpful for killing scabies mites while others reduce itching and redness. A combination of treatments may be necessary to eliminate all symptoms as well as the mites themselves. It is important for the patient to monitor himself as well as any household members being treated to ensure that infestation does not recur.

Sulfur Cream

Sulfur ointment has been used for centuries as a treatment for scabies.

A 5% to 10% ointment of sulfur mixed with petroleum jelly or cold cream is effective at eliminating scabies when applied for three consecutive nights and washed off 24 hours after the last treatment.

This is a particularly good option for children but people sensitive to sulfur should not use it. Side effects may include irritation and dry skin. Sulfur also has a strong odor, of course, and can stain bedding and clothing.

A doctor or naturopath should supervise treatment because of the potential for sensitivity in large doses in small children. A naturopath can also mix the solution or the patient can buy prepared sulfur applications that include other healing ingredients like tea tree oil, Aloe vera, zinc oxide and vitamin E. These medicaments are further discussed below in this section.

Tea Tree Oil – Melaleuca Oil: Six Treatments, Many Uses

Long appreciated for its antibacterial and antiseptic properties, tea tree oil is also helpful for killing scabies mites. The Menzies School of Public Health in Darwin, Australia has effectively used tea tree oil to treat scabies in Aboriginals found in remote areas where up to half of the population has chronic scabies infestation.

Applying tea tree oil to the skin soothes the itch of a scabies reaction while killing mites. Hence, this approach is a much better option than chemical treatments that prolong the itching.

Tea tree oil is an essential oil from the plant *Melaleuca alternifolia*, a species of tea tree found in Australia. Tea Tree oil is often used to treat acne, athlete's foot, yeast infections and psoriasis. Although creams, ointments, soaps and lotions containing tea tree oil are available, for best results only the pure essential oil should be used. It is for external use only. Tea tree oil should be kept from children and household animals.

When using tea tree oil to treat scabies, draw a warm bath and add 10 to 20 drops of tea tree oil to the water. Soak all infected areas, taking care to avoid contact with eyes or mouth. Rinse and dry thoroughly.

Pure tea tree oil may be applied directly to affected areas

with a cotton ball. Repeat this procedure once or twice a day for 2 to 3 weeks or until rash and discomfort disappear. Tea tree oil is especially helpful in treating sores on the face and scalp since it is much gentler than pharmaceutical methods of treatment that warn patients against facial use.

Patients may continue to use 5 to 10 drops of tea tree oil in a bath to prevent scabies outbreaks in the future.

One of the best sources of tea tree oil is from Melaleuca – 'The Wellness Company.' A direct-marketing company, Melaleuca offers a variety of the highest quality nutritional supplements, personal care products and environmentally conscious cleaning supplies. Melaleuca Oil is an essential oil that penetrates quickly and soothes irritated skin. As a bonus, the oil easily dissolves dirt and has a pleasantly agreeable scent. A natural antiseptic, it fights topical infection and is called "The First Aid Kit in a Bottle."

6 Properties, Many Applications
Each property in Melaleuca Oil meets a different need:

1. Naturally antiseptic: Melaleuca Oil's antibacterial properties help prevent topical infection at the first sign of trouble.

2. Gently soothes: Thanks to terpinene-4-ol, the "ahh" sensation of Melaleuca Oil stops the scratching, which helps skin heal faster.

3. Safely penetrates: Melaleuca Oil moves quickly to the source of the problem, even through

unbroken skin. Cineole, another key ingredient, helps the oil penetrate skin.

    4. Beneficially non-caustic: Melaleuca offers two grades of oil, - T36-C5 Melaleuca Oil, non-irritating for most skin types and T40-C3 Melaleuca Oil, for more sensitive skin. Skin will not feel raw after using Melaleuca Oil.

    5. Effectively solvent: Melaleuca Oil's natural solvency helps dissolve dirt and stains.

    6. Pleasantly aromatic: The fragrance of Melaleuca Oil comforts and soothes with its pleasing aroma (sometimes described as a combination of eucalyptus and nutmeg).

Melaleuca Oil is a natural remedy for minor skin irritations. With an affordable price, Melaleuca Oil offers a host of benefits. Order today to add T36-C5 or T40-C3 Melaleuca Oil as part of a complete medicine cabinet or first aid kit.

Aloe Vera

Aloe vera is one of the most highly touted natural remedies around. The gel-like fluid housed inside Aloe vera fronds speeds healing of all sorts of skin ailments from acne to burns.

Soothing to the skin, it is vitamin rich and one of the few plant sources of vitamin B-12. Aloe v. is used to treat skin conditions such as eczema, psoriasis and poison ivy, so it is a natural choice to help clear sores brought about by scabies.

Aloe v. will not kill scabies mites but does ease some symptoms. It is best combined with an anti-parasitic remedy such as tea tree oil or balsam of Peru.

If possible, it is best to use aloe directly from the plant. Aloe v. is a rather sensitive plant, so in frost zone regions it must be grown indoors. A bathroom is a prime location for aloe as it thrives on warmth and humidity.

To use aloe v., simply break off a small bit of one of the fronds, squeeze out the gel and apply it to the scabies sores. Aloe v. eases itching while healing sore spots.

Zinc Oxide

Zinc oxide is commonly found as an ingredient in sunscreens. It is helpful at blocking out harmful ultraviolet rays of the sun.

It is also protective of the skin in other ways. It can help clear up rashes and thus is useful in combination with other remedies for healing scabies.

Safe for people of all ages to use, zinc oxide can be tolerated in relatively large amounts. Over-the-counter preparations of zinc oxide are available to treat diaper rash. On scabies spots, use according to the manufacturer's instructions.

These products usually have other soothing ingredients like Aloe vera and beeswax so they have other uses other than relieving baby's diaper rash.

Vitamin E

Vitamin E is vital to the metabolism of cells and is thought to prevent free radicals in the body from causing damage to cells, which can in turn cause cancer and other ailments.

Wheat germ and other whole-wheat products are a great natural source of vitamin E. Most people who eat enough whole grains get a sufficient amount of vitamin E in their diet. People with Crohn's disease or cystic fibrosis may need to supplement their diet at all times with vitamin E. People with skin problems can use supplements or creams to speed healing and prevent scarring.

Creams and lotions containing vitamin E are the best choices for those with scabies. Using a cream with vitamin E can reduce itching and promote healing. Such creams are easy to find in most drug stores, or you can break open a gel cap of vitamin E and rub the gel on affected areas.

Again, vitamin E alone will not eliminate scabies but it can be helpful to reduce redness and itchiness associated with the ailment.

Balsam of Peru

Balsam of Peru, also sometimes seen as Peru Balsam, is an essential oil collected from trees found in El Salvador (it is processed in Peru, hence the name).

The oil has been used to treat eczema and arthritis. It can kill scabies because of its anti-parasitic properties. An amount of 10 to 30 drops should be given daily in a syrup solution (castor oil is a good choice) with an egg yolk added.

It is said to raise blood pressure, so those with hypertension may choose to avoid this approach.

Goldenseal

When used as a topical treatment, goldenseal can help fight infection. This is especially helpful when treating scabies because patients routinely contract infections when scratching itchy sores. However, it will not kill mites.

Goldenseal creams are commercially available. Some also include calendula, also known as marigold, which is thought to help heal skin and reduce scarring.

Goldenseal tea, especially in combination with Echinacea (another herbal remedy commonly used to boost the immune system) can also be helpful.

Tamanu Oil

Indigenous to Southeast Asia and Polynesia, the tamanu tree is known by many different names including ati, kamani and foraha. The tree produces a nut that, when cracked and dried, allows tamanu oil to develop.

The oil is pressed before bottling. It is beneficial for all sorts of skin ailments, including healing of wounds and scars. The oil can be applied pure or in a mixture with olive oil (which is also great for the skin) as needed. It is for external use only.

Garlic
Where would the world be without garlic? It is a versatile plant with both culinary and medicinal applications. Its uses have been studied and documented since the ancient Egyptians and Greeks.

Among the many properties of this wonder drug are its ability to lower blood pressure and cholesterol. Known as a strong anti-fungal and anti-parasitic herb, garlic's properties lends itself as treatment for scabies.

Taken internally, garlic will help kill scabies mites. Those afflicted with scabies can also pound a clove of garlic to extract the oil, which can be used alone or with olive oil, to rub on sores.

Rubbing garlic over the entire body is not recommended as it may produce dermatitis in some people.

Garlic is available in pill form, but it is best to use oil from real cloves rubbed on the skin for maximum anti-bacterial and anti-parasitic power.

Colloidal Silver
One of the most controversial natural remedies available today is colloidal silver. A reputed antibiotic cure-all and infection preventer, it is claimed to be effective against fungus, bacteria and viruses by disabling their oxygen metabolisms without harming the patient.

This was a common remedy as recently as the 1930s but fell out of favor when cheaper antibiotics (chemically produced by the pharmaceutical industry) came into favor.

Silver can be taken internally or applied directly from a spray bottle to affected areas such as scabies sores.

The treatment is controversial because of the proliferation of inferior products on the market. Many companies hawking the effectiveness of their colloidal silver sell impure products that are often ineffective.

Some worry about the accumulation of silver in the body due to chronic intakes of colloidal silver over a long period, as a dermatological condition known as argyria may occur. Yet many have found success using colloidal silver to treat everything from mouth sores, stuffy noses, and eye ailments to sores caused by scabies. It is even used as a deodorant because it is said to kill the bacteria that causes underarm odor.

Apply colloidal silver directly to scabies sores and burrows. It can be used undiluted twice a day. It does not sting or burn. It is especially helpful at preventing a secondary infection that could result from scratching scabies sores.

Black Walnut and Wormwood

Black walnut and wormwood are two herbal remedies that help the body fight parasitic infections. They are often found together in prepared tinctures and remedies for parasitic infections.

Black walnut hulls have long been used as a treatment for worms. They are full of iodine and tannins, which are antiseptic. They can help cleanse the blood and can be used to treat a variety of skin problems.

Wormwood is so named because it is a powerful defense against parasitic worms. It is also a general tonic and aids in proper digestion, so it is beneficial in a variety of ways when taken to treat scabies.

Neem Tree Leaf

A popular herb in Ayurvedic medicine, the neem tree is called the "wonder tree of India." Through the years, it has been used to treat infection, viruses and bacteria, burns, skin diseases and urinary disorders, among other ailments. Neem has even been used to treat malaria.

One of the chemical components of the tree has been found to be 95% effective as a pesticide and insecticide. The bark of the tree is used to eliminate worms and heal wounds, so it can also be helpful in getting rid of scabies and its sores.

Neem oil is a popular treatment for head lice and dandruff. The oil can be combined (10% to 90%) with another oil such as coconut or sesame oil and applied to the hair as a treatment for lice or dandruff. This treatment may also benefit those with scabies sores on the face or at the hairline.

The best part of the neem tree, however, is the leaves. Thought by practitioners of ayurvedic medicine to have an almost magical effect on the skin, the leaves are antifungal, antiseptic and anti-inflammatory and have been used to treat ringworm, eczema, acne and many other skin problems (Ayurveda is an Eastern system of health and wellness that has been practiced for more than 5,000 years.)

A scabies treatment that has proven to be quite effective involves neem tree leaves combined with turmeric in a 4:1 ratio by weight. Grind them into a paste, apply to the body and allow to dry. It should be washed off daily and repeated until symptoms are gone, usually within 3 to 5 days.

Those without access to a neem tree can purchase neem tree leaf to make this concoction. Add liquid such as olive oil to convert the ground herbs into a paste. Turmeric can also stain skin, clothing, etc., so use old clothes and linen that can be discarded before attempting this treatment.

Additional Helpful Herbs

Here are other herbal supplements that can be used to clear up scabies and associated itching and bumps.

• Gingko biloba is said to be helpful as an anti-oxidant and can be used as a cream to soothe scabies sores. Those on blood thinners should not use it.

• Kelp can be useful in restoring needed balance to a patient's mineral intake when recovering from an outbreak of scabies.

• Vitamin A is needed by the body to heal and reconstruct skin tissue once scabies sores have been eliminated.

• Evening primrose oil, which provides an essential fatty acid, is considered helpful for all sorts of skin disorders. Take by pill, 1,000 milligrams 3 times daily, with food. Vitamin E helps slow the breakdown of the acid, so look for products combining primrose oil with E.

• Sheep sorrel is an anti-parasitic found in anti-parasite tinctures with wormwood and black walnut.

• Cloves are great for detoxifying the body and are one of the few natural remedies known to kill parasite eggs in the body.

Suggested Natural Solution Steps
If diagnosed with scabies, for best results follow this quick and easy procedure for healing scabies naturally.

1. Bathe using warm water and 10 to 20 drops of tea tree essential oil.
Stay in the bath as long as desired, but 20 or 30 minutes is ideal. Make sure that the entire body from the neck down is immersed in water.

2. Towel dry and, using a cotton boll, apply pure

tea tree oil to the scabies sores. Apply Tea Tree oil to the sores 2 or 3 times daily until healed. Tea tree oil is an antiseptic that kills scabies mites, so be diligent with treatment. Continue bathing daily.

3. For severe itching, apply a lotion containing Aloe vera or use Aloe vera directly from the plant. Apply as often as needed to soothe itching. If buying a prepared Aloe vera lotion, look for one containing other healing ingredients, such as vitamin E, vitamin A, evening primrose oil, zinc oxide or goldenseal.

4. To increase anti-parasitic power, crush a glove of fresh garlic in a tablespoon of olive oil and rub the mixture only on the sores. Increasing the consumption of fresh garlic can help heal the body from the inside.

5. Wash all clothing and linens that all household members have contacted over the past week. Wash items for each family member separately and in hot water. Dry items in a clothes dryer, using the hottest setting. Repeat this process once treatment is complete for extra insurance against re-infestation.

6. Items that cannot be washed or fit in a washer or dryer may be sealed in a plastic bag and stored untouched for 7 days.

7. Use a lotion containing vitamin E to reduce itching and heal the skin.

Adding vitamin E to one's diet through supplements or foods (wheat germ and other whole grains) can also be helpful at speeding the healing of sores. Vitamin E is beneficial in metabolizing evening primrose oil. To increase the healing of skin, take evening primrose oil (1,000 milligrams taken with food 3 times daily) with vitamin E.

Parasite Detox

Another treatment for scabies that can be incredibly helpful and effective is known as a parasite cleanse. Cleanses have been used as a natural treatment for eradicating and curing a whole host of ailments since long before the advent of modern medicine.

Many common maladies prevalent today can be traced back to a need to cleanse the body of toxins. Toxins are substances found in the environment, from polluted air and water to the pesticides used in the food we eat and chemicals used to make household products that can accumulate in the body, causing harmful effects.

It is proven that if toxins are eliminated from the body, many illnesses will go away. Cleanses can be used to cure acne and other skin ailments, bowel problems, kidney problems and many other diseases and disorders - including scabies.

Dr. Hulda Clark is a naturopath who suggests that all diseases are caused by either parasites or pollution. Parasites can be eradicated through cleansing and pollutants can be avoided. Thus, all disease is avoidable and most can be cured through diligent cleansing.

As obviously scabies is caused by a parasite, doing a parasite cleanse can rid scabies infestations quickly. As with all other remedies suggested in this guide, all household members should be cleansed at the same time for optimal results. As in other remedies, linens and clothing should also be treated.

Dr. Clark's parasite cleanse involves herbs discussed in the last chapter: black walnut hulls, wormwood and cloves, herbs that provide powerful anti-parasitic protection. Clark claims that walnut hulls and wormwood will kill the adult parasites (scabies mites) while cloves kills the eggs.

All three herbs must be taken together for success. The black walnut hulls are ingested as a tincture, mixed in half a cup of water, and drunk slowly. Wormwood capsules with 200 to 300 milligrams of wormwood should be taken daily before a meal.

Clark advises against using cloves bought from grocery stores; because of processing and languishing on the shelf, they are ineffective. Buy herbal capsules that contain 500 milligrams of cloves and take before each meal.

The amount of tincture to take and the number of pills

to swallow vary each day, depending on program. She suggests following the protocol for continued good health, taking the herbs once a week for life after the first several days.

Other forms of cleanses and fasts that target bowel health can be helpful for eliminating parasites, including scabies, from the body. As a side benefit, these practices may resolve other health problems. However, the use of powerful anti-parasitic herbs such as wormwood, black walnut hulls and cloves makes cleansing much more effective at eliminating scabies. Of course, the inclusion of topical application of tea tree oil while using these herbs would likely lead to even quicker success at eliminating scabies.

Avoid Future Infections

Scabies mites can live on the human body for 2 to 5 days, so a clean environment is very important as part of treating scabies in order to prevent reinfection.

Several steps are needed to rid any lingering scabies mites in the home:

- Change linens immediately after applying treatment;

- Launder linens, all clothes, towels and washcloths used in the past week in hot water and dry in a dryer's hottest setting. Wash each family member's clothes separately and on the hottest setting for at least 10 minutes;

- Non-washable items such as shoes, stuffed animals, coats and other fabric items should be sealed in a plastic bag. They can be frozen in a - 4° Fahrenheit freezer for 12 hours or simply sealed and stored at room temperature for a week;

- Any creams, ointments or lotions used by an infected person in the week before treatment should be discarded. Cosmetics can be sealed in a plastic container and kept at room temperature for 2 weeks before using again;

- Vacuum carpeted floors and upholstered furniture. Keep furniture covered with a sheet or plastic for a week after treatment.

Following these protocols in addition to a treatment method discussed earlier should prevent any recurrence of scabies.

Lice and Bedbugs

While this publication is meant to be a guide to
scabies and its causes, effects and treatments, it
makes sense to mention other mites that cause
problems for humans: lice and bedbugs.

Facts about Lice

Lice are well known to anyone who has ever had
children. They are small insects - about the size of a
sesame seed and similar to scabies mites - usually found
in the hair. Like scabies, they pass quickly from person
to person, especially between prolonged contact of the
hair or when hairbrushes, ribbons or ponytail holders are
shared among infested and non-infested people.

If a child goes to school with lice, he will likely spread
the parasites among his classmates. Again, contracting
head lice comes from being in contact with an infected
person rather than personal hygiene. Once one child in a
classroom has lice, likely other children will become
infected, too. Conversely, once a family member gets lice,
it is likely that others in the family will also become
infected - especially those who share beds or bedrooms.

Lice are flightless insects and cannot jump. They are clear
when born and turn red or brown after feeding on the
human they infest. They have six legs and survive on
human blood.

Lice live about 30 days on a host, during which time a
female can lay about 100 eggs or nits. A female louse

must be present in order to have nits; one does not "catch nits." Eggs hatch in 7 to 10 days and lice become sexually mature 7 to 10 days later. Like scabies mites, they usually die within 24 hours after separation from a human host.

Besides head lice, there are also body lice, distinguished by their location on parts of the body other than hair. They often lay their eggs on the inside seams of clothing.

Pubic lice are also known as crab lice (since infestation in the pubic area is called "crabs"). Easily identifiable, they are a separate species of insect, distinct from lice that attach to the body and hair of the head.

Pubic lice are usually spread by sexual contact, although it is possible to contract them from an infected bedmate. If a child gets pubic lice, it is a strong indication that he or she is sexually active (or has been sexually abused).

Facts about Bed Bugs

Bedbugs used to be quite common from ancient times until as late as the 1950s. Use of the pesticide DDT eradicated much of the bedbug population, but the little critters have rebounded globally in recent years.

There are many theories for this resurgence. People are traveling more, including international travel, thus it is possible people are transporting bedbugs from areas where they are more prevalent to a country like the U.S. that has eradicated most of the native population.

The bait gels commonly used to fight bedbugs nowadays are not as effective as previous methods because bedbugs are not attracted to gel at room temperature; they search for warm bodies on which to feed.

Bedbugs are 1/8 to 1/4 inch in size and usually brown in color, although they appear redder after feeding on a human. They are commonly found in beds, thus the name. They like to hide in mattress tufts, under sheets, in the bed frame, even in little cracks between planks of a wood floor or sides of a picture frame.

As bedbugs develop, they go through five different stages, all of which require a diet of blood. It usually takes 5 to 10 minutes for a bedbug to sate its appetite. The whole process of development takes 6 to 8 weeks and the bugs live 6 to 12 months on average. After mating, a female bedbug can lay 2 or 3 eggs a day for the rest of her life. Eggs usually hatch in about 10 days.

They bite their human prey at night, often in the abdomen area. Blood on the bed sheets is the only way victims know that they have been bit. Soon after the bite, a red welt will appear. Bedbugs can lead to more severe health problems, especially in sensitive individuals.

Bedbugs can live a long time without feeding. They do not need constant human contact to survive, unlike scabies mites and lice. Hence, a bed that has not been slept in for some time is no protection against bedbugs.

It is much more difficult to eradicate bedbugs compared to

lice or scabies. This is because they do not remain on the victim's body after feeding and they can hide just about anywhere in a room. It is often suggested that infested mattresses be destroyed instead of trying to clean them because there are so many places for a bug to hide.

Washable materials can be treated in the same manner as a scabies infestation. Care must be taken to locate any possible hiding place in a room, including drawers, cracks in the floor, inside telephones, behind books - literally, any place a tiny bug could hide. Using a flashlight, slowly search all nooks and crannies in an infested room to find the critters.

These three insects – scabies mites, lice and bedbugs – are different but they affect people in similar ways. Likewise, they are traditionally treated in similar ways.

Most of the chemicals used on scabies can also treat lice, though they are often formulated in smaller concentrations and designed to be used as a rinse rather than a leave-on treatment.

Pyrethrum-derived products are popular choice for treating rooms that have been infested with bedbugs. You can spray everything in a room with this wonderful chemical and the bedbugs die, no matter where they are hiding.

Of course, those who have read the rest of this guide know that the above endorsement might not be such as good idea.

All the natural treatments listed above can be helpful for

eradicating lice and bedbugs as well as scabies, although the anti-parasitic remedies may not be as effective on bedbugs since bedbugs do not actually live on the victim's body. Everything mentioned as a treatment for the itch and redness of scabies mites and head lice can alleviate some of the pain and irritation caused by bedbug bites.

Boric acid is a good natural insecticide that has been used to kill cockroaches, Palmetto bugs, silverfish, termites and other notoriously resilient critters. It is deadly to all insects yet thought to be gentle enough to use around children. It is odorless and non-staining. Boric acid can be fatal if ingested in very large quantities (on par with table salt) but is generally thought to be safe if children are supervised around it.

Intriguing Facts about Scabies

- It is estimated that 300 million cases of scabies infestation occur each year around the world.

- Scabies have infested humans for around 2,500 years.

- Condoms do not prevent the transmission of scabies.

- An online search for scabies products retrieves more than 400,000 websites.

- Scabies is much more common in other countries outside of the United States. In fact, American foster parents are sometimes advised to beware of scabies in their newly adopted children.

- Scabiophobia is the psychological term for a fear of scabies.

- Taking a sauna regularly may be helpful in preventing future outbreaks of scabies.

- Bathing with diluted borax, enzyme solutions, lice shampoo or sulfur has also been suggested as ways to prevent a recurrence of scabies.

- **Do not** try to treat scabies with hard soaps, kerosene or laundry detergent.

Norwegian Scabies

Though most people are much more likely to be exposed to regular scabies compared to Norwegian scabies, it is worth taking a closer look at this serious manifestation.

Norwegian scabies, as noted earlier, is caused by the same mites that are associated with the more common form of scabies. The difference is that in Norwegian scabies, also known as crusted scabies, many more mites are infesting the body at any given time. Thus, the allergic reaction to the infestation is much more severe.

Instead of the standard acne-like bumps and itchy rashes of standard scabies, people with Norwegian scabies get large, crusty sores.

The first case of Norwegian scabies was seen in 1848, when it was thought to be a variation of leprosy. In 1851, it was identified as a variation of scabies and named for the country in which it was discovered.

Instead of 5 to 20 mites that might be present on a person with standard scabies, a person with Norwegian scabies will have thousands or even millions of mites in his or her body at any given time.

The difference between people who get standard scabies and those who get Norwegian scabies is due to their immune system. Healthy people tend to get the standard, less severe form of scabies, while those with compromised immune systems contract the more severe type.

Thus, it is more common in the elderly and those with weakened immune systems such as AIDS, lupus, multiple sclerosis or multiple chemical sensitivity.

Norwegian scabies can be difficult to diagnose because it looks like a rash that could arise from an allergic reaction or some other medical condition. Sometimes people who have this form of scabies will get a rash but it will not itch. Norwegian scabies seems to be more contagious than standard scabies in that, even when passed to someone who presents typical scabies symptoms; it tends to incubate for a shorter period before showing symptoms.

In addition, when scales of skin fall off from the flaky sores, these scales contain many mites, so there are more chances for them to migrate to another human with less contact.

Hence, it is possible to get scabies from a person with Norwegian scabies even without touching them or sharing articles of clothing or bedding with them. The mites cannot fly but they are much more likely to transmit via skin cells because there are so many mites involved in a Norwegian infestation.

Treatment for Norwegian scabies is the same as treatment for standard scabies, but one has to wonder how an already weak immune system will react to drugs that are essentially insecticides.

This is why it is so important to be informed about

potential natural cures for scabies. People who are already weak from other diseases will likely react poorly to the harsh medicines conventionally used to treat scabies.

Scabies and Community Health

Because of the ease of transmission among people who

share close quarters, it is particularly difficult to control an outbreak of scabies among people who live together in nursing homes or other institutions. Likewise, because of the close and often physical contact among children at day-care centers, those facilities are likely to become breeding grounds for scabies, just as they are for lice.

For that reason, it is particularly important that public health officials and staff at hospitals, clinics, nursing homes and daycare centers are educated about scabies. They should also have developed a plan for diagnosing and treating the patient or client population should an outbreak occur (or to have a plan for identifying scabies early so that it does not become an outbreak).

Everything said thus far about diagnosing and treating scabies is valid, whether it is one person with scabies or an entire floor of a nursing home. The difference is that treatments must occur on a much larger scale.

All of the bedding that infected patients have used must be washed, including communal items that may have been used by someone with scabies.

All visitors to an institution (or household, classroom, etc.) infected with scabies will need to be notified and treated, as well as their family and household members. As one may imagine, the circle of potentially affected people can become very wide very quickly. Regular record keeping will be helpful in determining who has been in the area and might have been infected.

Parents, children and family members of those living in nursing homes, assisted living facilities or other similar institution need to be educated about scabies and aware that such an infestation is possible. Keep an eye on your loved one for signs of infestation and be aware of what is going on in terms of hygiene in the facility.

A facility does not have to be unhygienic in order for scabies to be passed around but transmission is facilitated if, for instance, sheets are not being washed as often as they should or fabric items are shared between patients.

Those who work in such facilities without plans for dealing with scabies (or lice or any other contagious infestation or infection) should consider making this guide available to job supervisors and coworkers. A discussion needs to be started and plans formulated for addressing contagions such as scabies. See the resources section below that will assist in planning strategies.

Newsletter Bonus

**Sign up today to receive more helpful health
and wellness tips!
www.SparrowPublication.com**

www.ingramcontent.com/pod-product-compliance
Lightning Source LLC
Chambersburg PA
CBHW070325290526
45791CB00003B/1265